Table of Contents

ACUTE PANCREATITIS DIET COOKBOOK : RECOVERY PLAN AND DIETARY MEASURES

Pancreatitis is a disease in which your pancreas becomes inflamed.

Your pancreas helps you regulate the way that your body processes sugar. It also serves an important function in releasing enzymes and helping you digest food.

When your pancreas becomes swollen or inflamed, it cannot perform its function. This condition is called pancreatitis.

Because the pancreas is so closely tied to your digestive process, it's affected by what you choose to eat. In cases of acute pancreatitis, pancreas inflammation is often triggered by gallstones.

The pancreas is a large gland behind your stomach and next to your small intestine. Your pancreas does two main things:

- It releases powerful digestive enzymes into your small intestine to help you digest food.

- It releases insulin and glucagon into your bloodstream. These hormones help your body control how it uses food for energy.

Your pancreas can be damaged when digestive enzymes begin working before your pancreas releases them.

Types of Pancreatitis

The two forms of pancreatitis are acute and chronic.

Acute pancreatitis is sudden inflammation that lasts a short time. It can range from mild discomfort to a severe, life-threatening illness. Most people with acute pancreatitis recover completely after getting the right treatment. In severe cases, acute pancreatitis can cause bleeding, serious tissue damage, infection, and cysts. Severe pancreatitis can also harm other vital organs such as the heart, lungs, and kidneys.

Acute pancreatitis is caused when trypsin becomes activated within the pancreas. Trypsin is an enzyme that is produced in the pancreas and released into the intestines, where it breaks down proteins as part of the digestive system.

Trypsin is inactive until it has reached the intestines. If trypsin becomes activated inside the pancreas, it will start to digest the pancreas itself, leading to irritation and inflammation of the pancreas. This becomes acute pancreatitis.

Chronic pancreatitis is long-lasting inflammation. It most often happens after an episode of acute pancreatitis. Another top cause is drinking lots of alcohol for a long period of time. Damage to your pancreas from heavy alcohol use may not cause symptoms for many years, but then you may suddenly have severe pancreatitis symptoms.

The repeated bouts of acute pancreatitis eventually take their toll on the pancreas, causing permanent damage, which then becomes chronic pancreatitis.

Chronic pancreatitis is usually a complication of recurrent episodes of acute pancreatitis. These can lead to permanent damage in the pancreas.

There is also Idiopathic Chronic Pancreatitis which has no known cause or reason. Idiopathic chronic pancreatitis accounts for most of the remaining cases. Most cases of idiopathic chronic pancreatitis develop in people aged 10 to 20 years and those aged over 50 years.

Other much rarer cases include:

Autoimmune chronic pancreatitis, in which the person's own immune system attacks the pancreas.

Heredity pancreatitis, where patients have a genetic condition and are born with a faulty pancreas

Cystic fibrosis, another genetic condition that damages organs including the pancreas

Pancreatitis Symptoms

Pancreatitis can suddenly manifest itself and can be diagnosed as either mild, acute, or chronic pancreatitis. Mild pancreatitis may heal on its own without treatment but if left unchecked can progress to severe and life-threatening complications.

The signs and symptoms of pancreatitis are not the same for each person. Mild to acute cases of pancreatitis can have the following symptoms :

- Fever

- Higher heart rate

- Nausea and vomiting

- Swollen and tender belly

- Pain in the upper part of your belly that goes into your back. Eating may make it worse, especially foods high in fat.

It is advised to consult your doctor immediately should you feel persistent pain in the abdomen and if the pain keeps you from comfortably sitting down.

Pancreatitis Complications

Pancreatitis can have severe complications, including:

1. Diabetes, if there's damage to the cells that produce insulin

2. Infection of your pancreas

3. Kidney failure

4. Malnutrition, if your body can't get enough nutrients from the food you eat because of a lack of digestive enzymes

5. Pancreatic cancer

6. Pancreatic necrosis, when tissues die because your pancreas isn't getting enough blood

7. Problems with your breathing when chemical changes in your body affect your lungs

8. Pseudocysts, when fluid collects in pockets on your pancreas. They can burst and become infected.

Pancreatitis Diagnosis

To diagnose acute pancreatitis, your doctor tests your blood to measure two digestive enzymes: amylase and lipase. High levels of these two enzymes mean you probably have acute pancreatitis.

Other tests can include:

a. Pancreatic function test to find out whether your pancreas is making the right amounts of digestive enzymes

b. Ultrasound, CT scan, and MRI, which make images of your pancreas

c. ERCP, in which your doctor uses a long tube with a camera on the end to look at your pancreatic and bile ducts

d. Biopsy, in which your doctor uses a needle to remove a small piece of tissue from your pancreas to be studied

In some cases, your doctor may test your blood and poop to confirm the diagnosis. They may also do a glucose tolerance test to measure damage to the cells in your pancreas that make insulin.

PANCREATITIS TREATMENT

Treatment For Acute Pancreatitis

You'll probably need to stay in the hospital, where your treatment may include:

1) Antibiotics if your pancreas is infected

2) Intravenous (IV) fluids, given through a needle

3) Low-fat diet or fasting. You might need to stop eating so your pancreas can recover. In this case, you'll get nutrition through a feeding tube.

4) Pain medicine

If your case is more severe, your treatment might include:

a) ERCP to take out gallstones if they're blocking your bile or pancreatic ducts

b) Gallbladder surgery if gallstones caused your pancreatitis

c) Pancreas surgery to clean out fluid or dead or diseased tissue

Treatment For Chronic Pancreatitis

If you have chronic pancreatitis, you might need more treatments, including:

1. Insulin to treat diabetes

2. Pain medicine

3. Pancreatic enzymes to help your body get enough nutrients from your food

4. Surgery or procedures to relieve pain, help

with drainage, or treat blockages

Symptoms of Chronic Pancreatitis

The symptoms of chronic pancreatitis are similar to those of acute pancreatitis. But you may also have:

a. Constant pain in your upper belly that radiates to your back. This pain may be disabling.

b. Diarrhea and weight loss because your pancreas isn't releasing enough enzymes to break down food

c. Upset stomach and vomiting

PANCREATITIS CAUSES AND RISK FACTORS

Acute pancreatitis causes include:

- Autoimmune diseases

- Drinking lots of alcohol

- Infections

- Gallstones

- Medications

- Metabolic disorders

- Surgery

- Trauma

In up to 15% of people with acute pancreatitis, the cause is unknown.

Chronic pancreatitis causes include:

- Cystic fibrosis

- Family history of pancreas disorders

- Gallstones

- High triglycerides

- Longtime alcohol use

- Medications

In about 20% to 30% of cases, the cause of chronic pancreatitis is unknown. People with chronic pancreatitis are usually men between ages 30 and 40.

In cases of chronic pancreatitis, in which flare-ups recur over time, your diet might have a lot to do with the problem. Researchers are finding out more about foods you can eat to protect and even help to heal your pancreas.

Pancreatitis can also be genetic, or the symptom of an autoimmune reaction. In many cases of acute pancreatitis, the condition is triggered by a blocked bile duct or gallstones.

Obesity increases the risk for pancreatitis, so achieving and maintaining a healthy weight may help lower risk of developing pancreatitis. A healthy weight also lowers risk for gallstones, which are a common cause of pancreatitis.

OTHER TREATMENTS FOR PANCREATITIS

If your pancreas has been damaged by pancreatitis, a change in your diet will help you feel better. But it might not be enough to restore the function of the pancreas completely.

Your doctor may prescribe supplemental or synthetic pancreatic enzymes for you to take with every meal.

If you're still experiencing pain from chronic pancreatitis, consider alternative therapy such as yoga or acupuncture to supplement your doctor's prescribed pancreatitis treatment.

An endoscopic ultrasound or a surgery might be recommended as the next course of action if your pain continues

Besides making insulin, which your body uses to regulate blood sugar, a healthy pancreas produces enzymes that help your body digest and make use of the food you eat. If your pancreas becomes inflamed (pancreatitis), it has a harder time breaking down fat and isn't able to absorb as much nutrition. A pancreatitis diet takes this into account, prohibiting fatty foods and emphasizing choices that are nutrient-rich, especially those high in protein.

Changing how you eat, either temporarily or committing to a long-term pancreatitis diet, can help you manage your symptoms and prevent attacks, as well as keep you properly nourished despite your condition.

About 15% of people who have an episode of acute pancreatitis will have another. Chronic pancreatitis happens in closer to 5% of people.

The most common cause of chronic pancreatitis is alcohol abuse, accounting for approximately 80% of cases. Although diet does not directly cause pancreatitis (it can contribute to gallstones and increase lipid levels, both of which can lead to the condition, however), it can help treat symptoms and prevent future attacks in those who are diagnosed with the condition.

And the benefits go beyond comfort. A pancreatitis diet helps support an organ that's already functioning inefficiently, which is of great significance because a pancreas that becomes unable to contribute to insulin regulation can give way to developing diabetes.

Central to all of this is fat restriction. The less you consume, the less burden you put on your pancreas which, due to pancreatitis, is already challenged when it comes to metabolizing fat.

A 2013 study published in the journal Clinical Nutrition found that male patients with pancreatitis who ate a high-fat diet were more likely to have ongoing abdominal pain. They were also more likely to be diagnosed with chronic pancreatitis at a younger age.

Furthermore, a 2015 review of treatment guidelines developed by researchers in Japan found that patients with severe chronic pancreatitis benefitted from a very low-fat diet, but people with milder cases usually tolerated dietary fat (especially if they took digestive enzymes with meals).

If you have recurrent attacks of pancreatitis and continued pain, your doctor may have you experiment with your daily fat intake to see if your symptoms improve.

The pancreatitis diet's promotion of nutrient-dense foods also helps you thwart the possibility of malnourishment. One reason this can happen is that several key vitamins (A, D, and E) are fat-soluble; issues with fat digestion beget issues with properly absorbing these nutrients.

Being deficient in one or more fat-soluble vitamins comes with its own set of symptoms and health risks. For example, vitamin A deficiency can cause night blindness and vitamin D deficiency has been linked to an increased risk of osteoporosis (especially after menopause).

CHRONIC PANCREATITIS DOS AND DON'TS

Chronic pancreatitis results in over 122,000 visits to a doctor and 56,000 hospitalizations annually in the United States.

The pancreas produces important enzymes and hormones that help break down foods.

The following treatments are commonly recommended for chronic pancreatitis.

Lifestyle changes

People with chronic pancreatitis will need to undergo some lifestyle changes. These will include:

Stopping alcohol consumption: Giving up drinking will help prevent further damage to the pancreas. It will also contribute significantly towards relieving the pain. Some people may need professional help to quit alcohol.

Stopping tobacco use: Smoking is not a cause of pancreatitis, but it can accelerate the progression of the disease.

While the specifics of a pancreatitis diet plan will depend on your dietary needs and preferences, there are some general guidelines you can use as a starting point.

It's generally recommended that you avoid food choices that are:

a.)   High in fat

b.)   Heavily processed

c.)   Having lot of sugar

d.)   alcoholic

These may include the following food items

- Alcohol

- Baked goods (doughnuts, muffins, bagels, biscuits, croissants)

- Battered/fried fish and shellfish

- Butter, lard, vegetable oil, margarine, ghee

- Cake, pies, pastries

- Cheese, cream cheese, cheese sauce

- Cookies, brownies, candy

- Eggs with yolk

- Fatty cuts of red meat, organ meat

- Fried foods/fast food (stir-fried vegetables, fried rice, fried eggs, French fries)

- Ice cream, pudding, custards, milkshakes, smoothies with dairy

- Jams, jellies, preserves

- Lamb, goose, duck

- Milk-based coffee drinks

- Nut butters (peanut, almond)

- Nuts and seeds (in moderation as tolerated)

- Potato or corn chips

- Processed meat (sausage, hot dogs, lunchmeat)

- Refined white flour options (e.g., bread, pancakes, waffles, granola, cereal, crackers, pretzels)

- Refried beans, olives

- Store-bought salad dressing, mayo, creamy pasta sauces (Alfredo), tahini

- Whole milk, full-fat dairy products

- Soda, energy drinks

The guidelines for fat intake if you have pancreatitis vary. For example, the Digestive Health Center at Stanford University recommends patients with chronic pancreatitis limit fat intake to 30 to 50 grams per day, depending on how well it's tolerated.

Fat is still an important part of a balanced diet—you just may need to start paying more attention to and adjusting your intake of the kind of fat you eat.

For example, a type of fat called medium-chain triglycerides (MCTs) can be digested without any help from your pancreas. Coconut and coconut oil are naturally rich sources of MCTs, but it's also available in supplement form.

If your body is struggling to process healthy fats, your doctor might suggest you take digestive enzymes. These synthetic enzymes help make up for what your pancreas can't produce. They usually come in a capsule that you take when you eat.

WHAT TO EAT

Food choices to consider may include:

- Air-popped popcorn (without butter/oil), wheat or spelt pretzels

- Beans, lentils, legumes

- Coconut/palm kernel oil (for MCTs)

- Corn or whole-wheat tortillas

- Couscous, quinoa, whole wheat pasta

- Dairy-free milk alternatives (almond, soy, rice)

- Egg whites

- Fish (cod, haddock)

- Fresh/frozen/canned fruits and vegetables

- Fruit and vegetable juice without sugar or carbonation

- Herbal tea, decaffeinated coffee (with small amounts of honey or non-dairy creamer, if desired)

- Lean cuts of meat

- Low-fat or non-fat dairy products (cottage cheese, Greek yogurt)

- Low-fat sweets (graham crackers, ginger snaps, tea biscuits)

- Nutritional supplement drinks (Boost, Ensure)

- Poultry (turkey, chicken) without the skin

- Reduced sugar jams and jellies

- Rice

- Low-fat/fat-free clear soups and broth (avoid milk-based or creamy types)

- Spices and fresh herbs (as tolerated), salsa, tomato-based sauces

- Steel-cut oats, bran, farina, grits

- Sugar-free gelatin, ice pops

- Tofu, tempeh

- Tuna (canned in water not oil)

- Whole grain bread, cereals, and crackers

The Health Benefits of Digestive Enzymes

Approaches

There are two overall approaches to managing pancreatitis with your diet. You may find you need to use both, depending on whether you are having an attack of symptoms or trying to prevent inflammation.

When you're having acute pancreatitis symptoms, eating a limited diet of easily digested foods can be soothing.

If you are in the middle of an acute attack, your doctor may want you to be on a limited diet of soft foods until your body heals.

For most mild cases of pancreatitis, complete bowel rest or a liquid-only diet is not necessary. A 2016 review of clinical guidelines for treating acute pancreatitis found that a soft diet was safe for most patients who were unable to tolerate their typical diet due to pancreatitis symptoms.

When symptoms of pancreatitis are severe or there are complications, a feeding tube or other methods of artificial nutrition may be necessary.

Duration

While you may be able to return to a less restricted diet once you are feeling better, doing so can cause symptoms to return. If you tend to have recurrent bouts of pancreatitis, changing how you eat for the long-term can help prevent attacks while ensuring you're probably nourished and hydrated.

Fruits and vegetables

Choose produce with plenty of fiber, whether fresh or frozen. Canned fruits and vegetables can also work well, though you'll want to drain and rinse them to reduce the sugar/salt content. High-fat produce like avocados may be too rich for you to digest if you have pancreatitis. You'll also want to avoid cooking produce with butter and oils or topping it with creamy sauces.

Dairy

Choose low-fat or fat-free milk and yogurt or dairy-free alternatives such as almond, soy, and rice milk. Most types of cheese are high in fat, though lower-fat options like cottage cheese may not worsen your symptoms and can be a good source of protein.

Grains

For the most part, you'll want to build your pancreatitis diet around fiber-rich whole grains. The exception can be when you're having symptoms and your doctor advises you to eat a balanced diet, during which time you may find white rice, plain noodles, and white bread toast are easier to digest. Check the ingredients list carefully for cereals and granola, as these products can have added sugar and brands with nuts may be too high in fat if you have pancreatitis.

Protein

Look for low-fat sources of protein to include in your pancreatitis diet such as white fish and lean cuts of skinless poultry. Beans, legumes, and lentils, as well as grains like quinoa, also make easy and tasty protein-packed meals. Nuts and nut butters are rich plant-based protein sources, but the high fat content may contribute to pancreatitis symptoms.

Desserts

Rich sweets, especially those made from milk like ice cream and custards, are usually too rich for people with pancreatitis. Avoid high-sugar desserts like cakes, cookies, pastries, baked goods, and candy. Depending on how well your body can regulate blood sugar, it may be fine to add honey or a little sugar to tea or black coffee, or to occasionally eat a small piece of dark chocolate.

Beverages

Alcohol must be completely avoided. If caffeinated tea, coffee, and soft drinks contribute to symptoms, you may choose to limit or avoid them as well. In general, avoiding soda will help you cut back on sugar in your diet. If you continue to drink coffee, avoid milk-based drinks with sweetened syrups. Hydration is important and, as always, water is the best choice. Herbal tea, fruit and vegetable juices, and nutritional supplement drinks recommended by your doctor are a few other options.

Recommended Timing

If you have pancreatitis, you may find that you feel better adhering to a certain eating schedule. Try eating several small meals and snacks throughout the day instead of three large ones.

If you tend to feel full quickly, it can also be helpful to avoid eating and drinking at the same time. You may also feel better if you avoid combining certain foods or ingredients; take note of how you feel after meals and make adjustments as needed.

Cooking Tips

Avoid fried, sautéed, or stir-fried foods. Instead, try baking, grilling, roasting, boiling, and steaming. Fats like butter, lard, and oils are best avoided, though you may tolerate small amounts for cooking.

Certain spices may be irritating, but turmeric and ginger are tasty and have digestive benefits.

CONSIDERATIONS ON GENERAL NUTRITION

In some cases, people with pancreatitis try to prevent symptoms by restricting their diet on their own, which also contributes to malnutrition. While there are foods that can make pancreatitis worse, there are also plenty of nutritious foods that also promote digestive health and may help reduce inflammation.

For example, plant-based and lean sources of animal protein, whole grains, and fiber-rich produce provide key vitamins and minerals your body can use for energy without putting too much stress on your digestive system.

Fiber is an essential component of a healthy diet, but you may need to adjust your intake according to how you feel. If you're having acute pancreatitis symptoms, you may want to stick to a low-fiber diet until you're feeling better.

A nutritionist can help you make choices that manage your condition and keep you healthy.

Maintaining adequate nutrition is especially important in cases of severe pancreatitis, as the body's energy needs may actually increase.

Research has shown that when patients with pancreatitis are underweight or critically ill from infections like sepsis, the amount of energy their bodies use at rest (resting energy expenditure) can increase by up to 50%.

MODIFICATIONS AND DIETARY RESTRICTIONS

If you have other health conditions, you may need to adjust your pancreatitis diet to ensure you're getting the nutrition you need. It's important that you share any other diagnoses you have with your healthcare team and seek help devising a diet that both manages your pancreatitis and other issue(s).

For example, attacks of pancreatitis can occur during pregnancy. Your dietary needs will be different when you're pregnant or nursing, however, so your plan may need to be adjusted accordingly.

Nutrition is also an important consideration if you have another medical condition that affects your digestion. For example, if you have inflammatory bowel disease or cystic fibrosis, you may already have issues with malabsorption. Having gallbladder disease means you are more likely to have digestive symptoms.

If you also have diabetes, your pancreas is already working extra hard—or not working well at all. In this case, the decisions you make about what you eat and drink will have an even greater effect on your overall health.

Additionally, people who have high levels of triglycerides (hypertriglyceridemia) may have stricter parameters in terms of avoiding or limiting foods that are high in saturated fats.

Flexibility

If you're dining out and are not sure how much fat is in a particular dish you're considering, ask your server. You may be able to lower the fat content by asking for swaps or substitutions, or splitting a dish with someone.

Be sure to read labels when you shop at the grocery store. For the most part, you'll want to look for products that are low-fat and fat-free. These days, there are many, making the diet easier to follow. Remember, though: While nutrition labels list the amount of fat per serving, a package may contain more than one serving.

Support and Community Influence

If you're feeling frustrated by or disappointed about the need to change how you eat, it can be helpful to talk to other people who have been through what you're experiencing.

Joining an in-person or online support group is one way to connect with other people managing pancreatitis through diet. What works for them may not work for you, but sharing ideas and support one another can help you keep up your motivation.

Cost

If your doctor wants you to take nutritional supplements, you'll find the price of vitamins varies considerably based on type, brand, and dose.

If you develop exocrine pancreatic insufficiency and your doctor wants you to start pancreatic enzyme replacement therapy (PERT), this can be another added cost.

Much like nutritional and vitamin supplements, you may be able to find PERT capsules at most pharmacies and health food stores. The product you'll need to purchase will depend on the combination of enzymes and amount (units) your doctor wants you to take with each meal.

If you have health insurance, ask your doctor if they can prescribe vitamins, nutritional supplements, or PERT. Your insurance may cover part or all of the cost. However, with PERT, coverage may be limited based on FDA approval.

Pain Management

Treatment should not only focus on helping ease the pain symptoms, but also depression which is a common consequence of long-term pain.

Doctors will usually use a step-by-step approach, in which mild painkillers are prescribed, gradually becoming stronger until pain becomes manageable.

POSSIBLE COMPLICATIONS

The pancreas may stop producing insulin if the damage is extensive. The individual is likely to have developed diabetes type 1.

Regular insulin treatment will become part of the treatment for the rest of the person's life. Diabetes type 1 caused by chronic pancreatitis involves injections, not tablets, because most likely the digestive system will not be able to break them down.

Constant or recurring pain may cause anxiety, irritability, stress, and depression.

There are several ways in which chronic pancreatitis can develop and become more harmful to a person's wellbeing.

Stress, Anxiety, and Depression

The disease may have an effect on the patient's psychological and emotional well being. Constant or recurring pain, which is often severe, may cause distress, anxiety, irritability, stress, and depression.

It is important for patients to tell their doctors if they are emotionally or psychologically affected. If there is a support group in your area, being able to talk to people who share the same condition may help you feel less isolated and more able to cope.

Pseudocyst

This is a collection of tissue, fluid, debris, pancreatic enzymes, and blood in the abdomen, caused by leakage of digestive fluids escaping from a faulty pancreatic duct.

Pseudocysts do not usually cause any health problems. However, sometimes they can become infected, cause blockage to part of the intestine, or rupture and cause internal bleeding. If this happens, the cyst will have to be surgically drained.

Pancreatic Cancer

Even though pancreatic cancer is more common among patients with chronic pancreatitis, the risk is only 1 in 500.

SURGERY

Severe chronic pain sometimes does not respond to painkilling medications. The ducts in the pancreas may have become blocked, causing an accumulation of digestive juices which puts pressure on them, causing intense pain. Another cause of chronic and intense pain could be inflammation of the head of the pancreas.

Several forms of surgery may be recommended to treat more severe cases.

1.   Endoscopic surgery

A narrow, hollow, flexible tube called an endoscope is inserted into the digestive system, guided by ultrasound. A device with a tiny, deflated balloon at the end is threaded through the endoscope. When it reaches the duct, the balloon is inflated, thus widening the duct. A stent is placed to stop the duct from narrowing back.

2.   Pancreas Resection

The head of the pancreas is surgically removed. This not only relieves the pain caused by inflammation irritating the nerve endings, but it also reduces pressure on the ducts. Three main techniques are used for pancreas resection:

a. **The Beger procedure**: This involves resection of the inflamed pancreatic head with careful sparing of the duodenum, the rest of the pancreas is reconnected to the intestines.

b. **The Frey procedure**: This is used when the doctor believes pain is being caused by both inflammation of the head of the pancreas as well as the blocked ducts. The Frey procedure adds a longitudinal duct decompression to the pancreatic head resection – the head of the pancreas is surgically removed, and the ducts are decompressed by connecting them directly to the intestines.

c. **Pylorus - sparing pancreaticoduodenectomy (PPPD):** The gallbladder, ducts, and the head of the pancreas are all surgically removed. This is only done in very severe cases of intense chronic pain where the head of the pancreas is inflamed, and the ducts are also blocked. This is the most effective procedure for reducing pain and conserving pancreas function. However, it has the highest risk of infection and internal bleeding.

3.   Total Pancreatectomy

This involves the surgical removal of the whole pancreas. It is very effective in dealing with the pain. However, a person who has had a total pancreatectomy will be dependent on treatment for some of the vital functions of the pancreas, such as the release of insulin.

4. Autologous Pancreatic Islet Cell Transplantation (APICT)

During the total pancreatectomy procedure, a suspension of isolated islet cells is created from the surgically removed pancreas and injected into the portal vein of the liver. The islets cells will function as a free graft in the liver and will produce insulin.

PREVENTION

Patients with acute pancreatitis significantly reduce their risk of developing chronic pancreatitis if they give up drinking alcohol. This is especially the case for patients who drink heavily and regularly.

The same enzymes that help with digestion can sometimes injure the pancreas and cause irritation. This irritation can be short-term or long-term.

Certain foods may make abdominal pain caused by pancreatitis worse. It is important to choose foods that will not make symptoms worse and cause discomfort while recovering from pancreatitis.

PANCREATITIS RECOVERY DIET

Taking dietary measures to reduce the effects of pancreatitis are vital.

The pancreas is involved in digestion, but pancreatitis can impair this function. This means that people with the disease will have difficulty digesting many foods.

Rather than three large meals a day, people with pancreatitis will be advised instead to consume six small meals. It is also better to follow a low-fat diet.

Managing the diet during pancreatitis aims to achieve four outcomes:

a. Reducing the risk of malnutrition and shortages of certain nutrients

b. Avoiding high or low blood sugar

c. Managing or preventing diabetes, kidney disease, and other complications

d. Decreasing the likelihood of an acute flare-up of pancreatitis

A diet plan will either be drawn up by the doctor, or the patient may be referred to a qualified dietitian. The plan is based on the current levels of nutrients in the blood shown in diagnostic testing.

Meal plans will generally involve food sources that are high in protein and have dense nutritional content. These are likely to include whole grains, vegetables, fruits, low-fat dairy products, and lean protein sources, such as boneless chicken and fish.

If you're recovering from acute or chronic pancreatitis, avoid drinking alcohol. If you smoke, you'll also need to quit. Focus on eating a low-fat diet that won't tax or inflame your pancreas.

You should also stay hydrated. Keep an electrolyte beverage or a bottle of water with you at all times.

If you've been hospitalized due to a pancreatitis flare-up, your doctor will probably refer you to a dietitian to help you learn how to change your eating habits permanently.

People with chronic pancreatitis often experience malnutrition due to their decreased pancreas function. Vitamins A, D, E, and K are most commonly found to be lacking as a result of pancreatitis.

This book gives you a day sample menu on pancreatitis diet and a 7-day pancreatitis meal plan you can follow to recover from acute pancreatitis.

DIET TIPS

Always check with your doctor or dietician before changing your eating habits when you have pancreatitis. Here are some tips they might suggest:

Eat between six and eight small meals throughout the day to help recover from pancreatitis. This is easier on your digestive system than eating two or three large meals.

Use MCTs as your primary fat since this type of fat does not require pancreatic enzymes to be digested. MCTs can be found in coconut oil and palm kernel oil and is available at most health food stores.

Avoid eating too much fiber at once, as this can slow digestion and result in less-than-ideal absorption of nutrients from food. Fiber may also make your limited amount of enzymes less effective.

Take a multivitamin supplement to ensure that you're getting the nutrition you need. You can find a great selection of multivitamins here.

WHAT TO EAT IF YOU HAVE PANCREATITIS

To get your pancreas healthy, focus on foods that are rich in protein, low in animal fats, and contain antioxidants. Try lean meats, beans and lentils, clear soups, and dairy alternatives (such as flax milk and almond milk). Beans and lentils may be recommended for a pancreatitis diet because of their high fiber content. Your pancreas won't have to work as hard to process these.

Research suggests that some people with pancreatitis can tolerate up to 30 to 40% of calories from fat when it's from whole-food plant sources or medium-chain triglycerides (MCTs). Others do better with much lower fat intake, such as 50 grams or less per day.

Spinach, blueberries, cherries, and whole grains can work to protect your digestion and fight the free radicals that damage your organs.

If you're craving something sweet, reach for fruit instead of added sugars since those with pancreatitis are at high risk for diabetes.

Consider cherry tomatoes, cucumbers and hummus, and fruit as your go-to snacks. Your pancreas will thank you.

WHAT NOT TO EAT IF YOU HAVE PANCREATITIS

Foods to limit include:

- red meat
- organ meats
- fried foods
- fries and potato chips
- mayonnaise
- margarine and butter
- full-fat dairy

- pastries and desserts with added sugars

- beverages with added sugars

If you're trying to combat pancreatitis, avoid trans-fatty acids in your diet.

Fried or heavily processed foods, like french fries and fast-food hamburgers, are some of the worst offenders. Organ meats, full-fat dairy, potato chips, and mayonnaise also top the list of foods to limit.

Cooked or deep-fried foods might trigger a flare-up of pancreatitis. You'll also want to cut back on the refined flour found in cakes, pastries, and cookies. These foods can tax the digestive system by causing your insulin levels to spike.

SAMPLE ONE DAY MENU

Breakfast

Scrambled eggs with spinach, (use egg whites only)

1 slice whole-wheat toast + 1 tbsp fruit compote/preserve

Black coffee or tea

AM Snack

An apple + tea or an Avocado smoothie

Lunch

Red rice and beans

1 pc Tortilla

3 oz Chicken breast, grilled

Salsa, guacamole

PM Snack

Whole wheat crackers, thins

1 banana

Water or Almond milk tea with chia seeds

Dinner

Green Salad with Grilled Shrimp + balsamic dressing

Fresh fruit juice.

In the meal plan are recipes for breakfast, lunch and dinner.

7 DAY PANCREATITIS MEAL PLAN

	Breakfast	**Lunch**	**Dinner**
Monday	Banana Yogurt Pots	Cannellini Bean Salad	Quick Moussaka
Tuesday	Tomato and Watermelon Salad	Edgy Veggie Wraps	Spicy Tomato Baked Eggs
Wednesday	Blueberry Oats Bowl	Carrot, Orange and	Salmon with Potatoes and Corn Salad

		Avocado Salad	
Thursday	Banana Yogurt Pots	Mixed Bean Salad	Spiced Carrot and Lentil Soup
Friday	Tomato and Watermelon Salad	Panzanella Salad	Med Chicken, Quinoa and Greek Salad
Saturday	Blueberry Oats Bowl	Quinoa and Stir Fried Veg	Grilled Vegetables with Bean Mash
Sunday	Banana Yogurt Pots	Moroccan Chickpea Soup	Spicy Mediterranean Beet Salad

Snacks are recommended between meal times.

Some good snacks include:

- A handful of nuts or seeds

- A piece of fruit

- Carrots or baby carrots

- Berries or grapes

DAY 1: MONDAY

BREAKFAST: Banana Yogurt Pots

Nutrition:

Calories – 236

Protein – 14g

Carbs – 32g

Fat – 7g

Prep time: 5 minutes

Ingredients (for 2 people)

- 225g Greek yogurt

- 2 bananas, sliced into chunks

- 15g walnuts, toasted and chopped

INSTRUCTIONS

Place some of the yogurt into the bottom of a glass. Add a layer of banana, then yogurt and repeat. Once the glass is full, scatter with the nuts.

LUNCH: Cannellini Bean Salad

Nutrition

Calories – 302

Protein – 20g

Carbs – 54g

Fat – 0g

Prep time: 5 minutes

Ingredients (for 2 people)

- 600g cans cannellini beans
- 70g cherry tomatoes, halved
- ½ red onion, thinly sliced
- ½ tbsp red wine vinegar
- small bunch basil, torn

INSTRUCTIONS

Rinse and drain the beans and mix with the tomatoes, onion and vinegar. Season, then add basil just before serving.

DINNER: Quick'n'Easy Moussaka

Nutrition

Calories – 577

Protein – 27g

Carbs – 46g

Fat – 27g

Prep time + cook time: 30 minutes

Ingredients (for 2 people)

- 1 tbsp extra virgin olive oil

- ½ onion, finely chopped

- 1 garlic clove, finely chopped

- 250g lean beef mince

- 200g can chopped tomatoes

- 1 tbsp tomato purée

- 1 tsp ground cinnamon

- 200g can chickpeas

- 100g pack feta cheese, crumbled

- Mint (fresh preferable)

- Brown bread, to serve

INSTRUCTIONS

Heat the oil in a pan. Add the onion and garlic and fry until soft. Add the mince and fry for 3-4 minutes until browned.

Tip the tomatoes into the pan and stir in the tomato purée and cinnamon, then season. Leave the mince to simmer for 20 minutes. Add the chickpeas halfway through.

Sprinkle the feta and mint over the mince. Serve with toasted bread.

DAY 2: TUESDAY

BREAKFAST: Tomato and Watermelon Salad

Nutrition

Calories – 177

Protein – 5g

Carbs – 13g

Fat – 13g

Prep time + cook time: 5 minutes

Ingredients (for 2 people)

- 1 tbsp olive oil
- 1 tbsp red wine vinegar
- ¼ tsp chilli flakes
- 1 tbsp chopped mint
- 120g tomatoes, chopped

- 250g watermelon, cut into chunks

- 50g feta cheese, crumbled

INSTRUCTIONS

For the dressing, Mix the oil, vinegar, chilli flakes and mint and then season.

Put the tomatoes and watermelon into a bowl. Pour over the dressing, add the feta, then serve.

LUNCH: Edgy Veggie Wraps

Nutrition

Calories – 310

Protein – 11g

Carbs – 39g

Fat – 11g

Prep time + cook time: 10 minutes

Ingredients (for 2 people)

100g cherry tomatoes

1 cucumber

6 Kalamata olives

2 large wholemeal tortilla wraps

50g feta cheese

2 tbsp houmous

INSTRUCTIONS

Chop the tomatoes, cut the cucumber into sticks,

split the olives and remove the stones.

Heat the tortillas.

Spread the houmous over the wrap. Put the vegetable mix in the middle and roll up.

DINNER: Spicy Tomato Baked Eggs

Nutrition

Calories – 417

Protein – 19g

Carbs – 45g

Fat – 17g

Prep time + cook time: 25 minutes

Ingredients (for 2 people)

- 1 tbsp olive oil

- 2 red onions, chopped

- 1 red chilli, deseeded & chopped

- 1 garlic clove, sliced

- small bunch coriander, stalks and leaves chopped separately

- 800g can cherry tomatoes

- 4 eggs

- brown bread, to serve

INSTRUCTIONS

Heat the oil in a frying pan with a lid, then cook the onions, chilli, garlic and coriander stalks for 5 minutes until soft. Stir in the tomatoes, then simmer for 8-10 minutes.

Using the back of a large spoon, make 4 dips in the sauce, then crack an egg into each one. Put a lid on the pan, then cook over a low heat for 6-8 mins, until the eggs are done to your liking. Scatter with the coriander leaves and serve with bread.

DAY 3: WEDNESDAY

BREAKFAST: Blueberry Oats Bowl

Nutrition

Calories – 235

Protein – 13g

Carbs – 38g

Fat – 4g

Prep time + cook time: 10 minutes

Ingredients (for 2 people)

- 60g porridge oats

- 160g Greek yogurt

- 175g blueberries

- 1 tsp honey

INSTRUCTIONS

Put the oats in a pan with 400ml of water. Heat and stir for about 2 minutes. Remove from the heat and add a third of the yogurt.

Tip the blueberries into a pan with the honey and 1 tbsp of water. Gently poach until the blueberries are tender.

Spoon the porridge into bowls and add the remaining yogurt and blueberries.

LUNCH: Carrot, Orange and Avocado Salad

Nutrition

Calories – 177

Protein – 5g

Carbs – 13g

Fat – 13g

Prep time + cook time: 5 minutes

Ingredients (for 2 people)

- 1 orange, plus zest and juice of 1

- 2 carrots, halved lengthways and sliced with a peeler

- 35g bag rocket/arugala

- 1 avocado, stoned, peeled and sliced

- 1 tbsp olive oil

INSTRUCTIONS

Cut the segments from 1 of the oranges and put in a bowl with the carrots, rocket and avocado. Whisk together the orange juice, zest and oil. Toss through the salad, and season.

DINNER: Salmon with Potatoes and Corn Salad

Nutrition

Calories – 479

Protein – 43g

Carbs – 27g

Fat – 21g

Prep time + cook time: 30 minutes

Ingredients (for 2 people)

- 200g baby new potatoes

- 1 sweetcorn cob

- 2 skinless salmon fillets

- 60g tomatoes

- 1 tbsp red wine vinegar

- 1 tbsp extra-virgin olive oil

- 1 shallot, finely chopped

- 1 tbsp capers, finely chopped

- handful basil leaves

INSTRUCTIONS

Cook potatoes in boiling water until tender, adding corn for final 5 minutes. Drain & cool.

For the dressing, mix the vinegar, oil, shallot, capers, basil & seasoning.

Heat grill to high. Rub some dressing on salmon & cook, skinnedside down, for 7-8 minutes. Slice tomatoes & place on plate. Slice the potatoes, cut the corn from the cob & add to plate. Add the salmon & drizzle over the remaining dressing.

DAY 4: THURSDAY

BREAKFAST: Banana Yogurt Pots

Lunch: Mixed Bean Salad

Nutrition

Calories – 240

Protein – 11g

Carbs – 22g

Fat – 12g

Prep time + cook time: 10 minutes

Ingredients (for 2 people)

- 145g jar artichoke heart in oil

- ½ tbsp sundried tomato paste

- ½ tsp red wine vinegar

- 200g can cannellini beans, drained and rinsed

- 150g pack tomatoes, quartered handful Kalamata black olives

- 2 spring onions, thinly sliced on the diagonal

- 100g feta cheese, crumbled

INSTRUCTIONS

Drain the jar of artichokes, reserving 1-2 tbsp of oil. Add the oil, sun-dried tomato paste and vinegar and stir until smooth. Season to taste.

Chop the artichokes and tip into a bowl. Add the cannellini beans, tomatoes, olives, spring onions and half of the feta cheese. Stir in the artichoke oil mixture and tip into a serving bowl. Crumble over the remaining feta cheese, then serve.

DINNER: Spiced Carrot and Lentil Soup

Nutrition

Calories – 238

Protein – 11g

Carbs – 34g

Fat – 7g

Prep time + cook time: 25 minutes

Ingredients (for 2 people)

- 1 tsp cumin seeds

- pinch chilli flakes

- 1 tbsp olive oil

- 300g carrots, washed and coarsely grated (no need to peel)

- 70g split red lentils

- 500ml hot vegetable stock (from a cube is fine)

- 60ml milk

- Greek yogurt, to serve

INSTRUCTIONS

Heat a large saucepan and dry fry the cumin seeds and chilli flakes for 1 minute. Scoop out about half of the seeds with a spoon and set aside. Add the oil, carrot, lentils, stock and milk to the pan and bring to the boil. Simmer for 15 minutes until the lentils have swollen and softened.

Whizz the soup with a stick blender or in a food processor until smooth. Season to taste and finish with a dollop of Greek yogurt and a sprinkling of the reserved toasted spices.

DAY 5: FRIDAY

BREAKFAST: Tomato and Watermelon Salad

Lunch: Panzanella Salad

Nutrition

Calories – 452

Protein – 6g

Carbs – 37g

Fat – 25g

Prep time + cook time: 10 minutes

Ingredients (for 2 people)

- 400g tomatoes

- 1 garlic clove, crushed

- 1 tbsp capers, drained and rinsed

- 1 ripe avocado, stoned, peeled and chopped

- 1 small red onion, very thinly sliced

- 2 slices of brown bread

- 2 tbsp olive oil

- 1 tbsp red wine vinegar

- small handful basil leaves

INSTRUCTIONS

Chop the tomatoes and put them in a bowl. Season well and add the garlic, capers, avocado and onion. Mix well and set aside for 10 minutes.

Meanwhile, tear the bread into chunks and place in a bowl. Drizzle over half of the olive oil and half of the vinegar. When ready to serve, scatter tomatoes and basil leaves and drizzle with remaining oil and vinegar. Stir before serving.

DINNER: Med Chicken, Quinoa and Greek Salad

NUTRITION

Calories – 473

Protein – 36g

Carbs – 57g

Fat – 25g

Prep time + cook time: 20 minutes

Ingredients (for 2 people)

- 100g quinoa

- ½ red chilli, deseeded and finely chopped

- 1 garlic clove, crushed

- 200g chicken

- 1 tbsp extra-virgin olive oil

- 150g tomato, roughly chopped

- handful pitted black kalamata olives

- ½ red onion, finely sliced

- 50g feta cheese, crumbled

- small bunch mint leaves, chopped

- juice and zest ½ lemon

INSTRUCTIONS

Cook the quinoa following the pack instructions, then rinse in cold water and drain thoroughly.

Meanwhile, toss the chicken fillets in the olive oil with some seasoning, chilli and garlic. Lay in a hot pan and cook for 3-4 minutes each side or until cooked through. Transfer to a plate and set aside

Next, tip the tomatoes, olives, onion, feta and mint into a bowl. Toss in the cooked quinoa. Stir through the remaining olive oil, lemon juice and zest, and season well. Serve with the chicken on top.

DAY 6: SATURDAY

BREAKFAST: Blueberry Oats Bowl

Lunch: Quinoa and Stir Fried Veg

Nutrition

Calories – 473

Protein – 11g

Carbs – 56g

Fat – 25g

Prep time + cook time: 30 minutes

Ingredients (for 2 people)

- 100g quinoa

- 3 tbsp olive oil

- 1 garlic clove, finely chopped

- 2 carrots, cut into thin sticks

- 150g leek, sliced

- 150g broccoli, cut into small florets

- 50g tomatoes

- 100ml vegetable stock

- 1 tsp tomato purée

- juice ½ lemon

INSTRUCTIONS

Cook the quinoa according to pack instructions. Meanwhile, heat 3 tbsp of the oil in a pan, then add the garlic and quickly fry for 1 minute. Throw in the carrots, leeks and broccoli, then stir-fry for 2 minutes until everything is glistening.

Add the tomatoes, mix together the stock and tomato purée, then add to the pan. Cover and cook for 3 minutes. Drain the quinoa and toss in the remaining oil and lemon juice. Divide between warm plates and spoon the vegetables on top.

DINNER: Grilled Vegetables with Bean Mash

Nutrition

Calories – 314

Protein – 19g

Carbs – 33g

Fat – 16g

Prep time + cook time: 40 minutes

Ingredients (for 2 people)

- 1 tbsp olive oil

- 1 tbsp red wine vinegar

- ¼ tsp chilli flakes

- 1 tbsp chopped mint

- 120g tomatoes, chopped

- 250g watermelon, cut into chunks

- 50g feta cheese, crumbled

INSTRUCTIONS

Heat the grill. Arrange the vegetables over a grill pan & brush lightly with oil. Grill until lightly browned, turn them over, brush again with oil, then grill until tender.

Meanwhile, put the beans in a pan with garlic and stock. Bring to the boil, then simmer, uncovered, for 10 minutes. Mash roughly with a potato masher. Divide the vegetables and mash between 2 plates, drizzle over oil and sprinkle with black pepper and coriander.

DAY 7: SUNDAY

BREAKFAST: Banana Yogurt Pots

LUNCH: Moroccan Chickpea Soup

Nutrition

Calories – 408

Protein – 15g

Carbs – 63g

Fat – 11g

Prep time + cook time: 25 minutes

Ingredients (for 2 people)

- 1 tbsp olive oil

- ½ medium onion, chopped

- 1 celery sticks, chopped

- 1 tsp ground cumin

- 300ml hot vegetable stock

- 200g can chopped tomatoes

- 200g can chickpeas, rinsed and drained

- 50g frozen broad beans

- zest and juice ½ lemon

- coriander & bread to serve

INSTRUCTIONS

Heat the oil in a saucepan, then fry the onion and celery for 10 minutes until softened. Add the cumin and fry for another minute.

Turn up the heat, then add the stock, tomatoes, chickpeas and black pepper. Simmer for 8 minutes. Add broad beans and lemon juice and cook for a further 2 minutes. Top with lemon zest and coriander.

DINNER: Spicy Mediterranean Beet Salad

NUTRITION

Calories – 548

Protein – 23g

Carbs – 58g

Fat – 20g

Prep time + cook time: 40 minutes

Ingredients (for 2 people)

- 8 raw baby beetroots, or 4 medium, scrubbed

- ½ tbsp za'atar

- ½ tbsp sumac

- ½ tbsp ground cumin

- 400g can chickpeas, drained and rinsed

- 2 tbsp olive oil

- ½ tsp lemon zest

- ½ tsp lemon juice

- 200g Greek yogurt

- 1 tbsp harissa paste

- 1 tsp crushed red chilli flakes

- mint leaves, chopped, to serve

INSTRUCTIONS

Heat oven to 220C/200C fan/ gas 7. Halve or quarter beetroots depending on size. Mix spices together. On a large baking tray, mix chickpeas and beetroot with the oil. Season with salt & sprinkle over the spices. Mix again. Roast for 30 minutes.

While the vegetables are cooking, mix the lemon zest and juice with the yogurt. Swirl the harissa through and spread into a bowl. Top with the beetroot & chickpeas, and sprinkle with the chilli flakes & mint.

FINAL THOUGHT

Pancreatitis can be a painful and frustrating condition, especially when it becomes chronic. There isn't a single pancreatitis diet that works for everyone, but diet can have a big impact on how you feel. Know that finding the right plan for you can take time, and work with your doctor, a registered dietician, and/or nutritionist to fine-tune a pancreatic diet that meets your needs.

Nutrition plays a vital role in treating pancreatitis. The impact of this disease in patients can be devastating if left unmanaged. Once a patient has been diagnosed with pancreatitis, proper diet and nutrition is the main goal for pancreatitis management to help with the impact of the disease in the patient. These specific goals are crucial in the treatment and management of the disease.